Nancy L. Morse BSc CNPA

Attention-Deficit Disorder

Natural Alternatives to Drug Therapy

D0040316

alive books

Vancouver
Canada

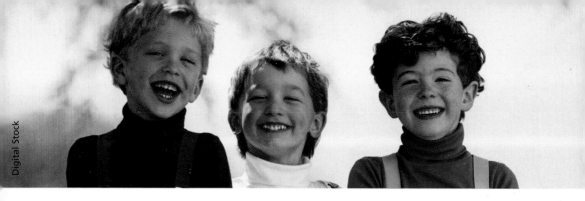

Digital Stock

Contents

Note: Conversions in this book (from imperial to metric) are not exact. They have been rounded to the nearest measurement for convenience. Exact measurements are given in imperial. The recipes in this book are by no means to be taken as therapeutic. They simply promote the philosophy of both the author and *alive* books in relation to whole foods, health and nutrition, while incorporating the practical advice given by the author in the first section of the book.

Recipes

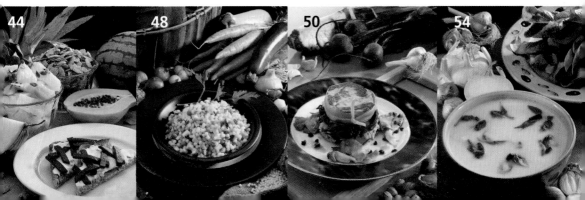

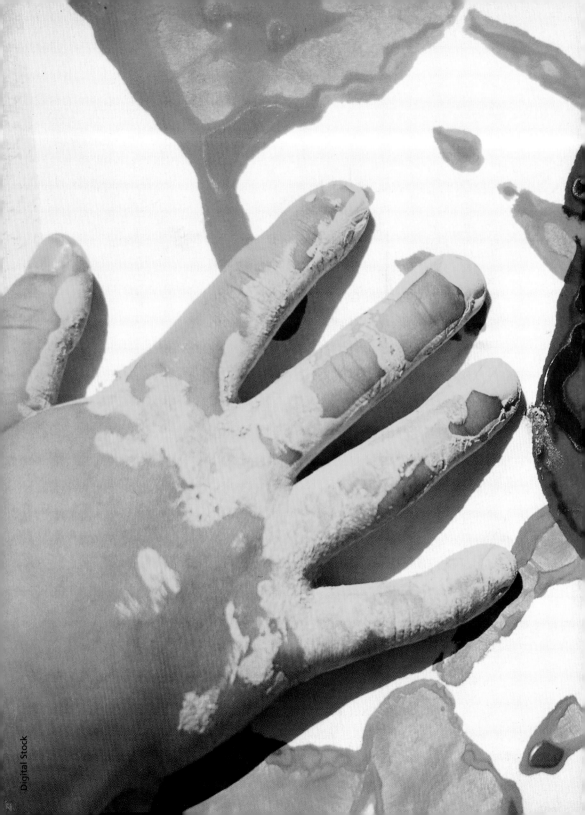

**There are options
–natural options–
available to treat attention
and learning disorders.**

Introduction . . . .

Learning disorders, especially attention-deficit disorder (ADD), attention-deficit hyperactivity disorder (ADHD), hyperactivity, dyslexia, dyspraxia and combinations of these problems, are reaching epidemic proportions in Western societies. Probable causes of these conditions range from lifestyle to environmental to genetic influences, and combinations of these factors, but no one knows for sure why these problems develop. Two things are certain, however: the conditions do exist and there are ways to help minimize the problems associated with them.

Considering...
- the number of people being diagnosed with ADD/ADHD;
- the obvious damaging effects of the current drug treatments;
- that the majority of patients being treated are children;
- that they are being treated for prolonged periods of time;
- and that conventional drugs have uncertain long-terms effects

There is hope for those affected by attention and learning disorders.

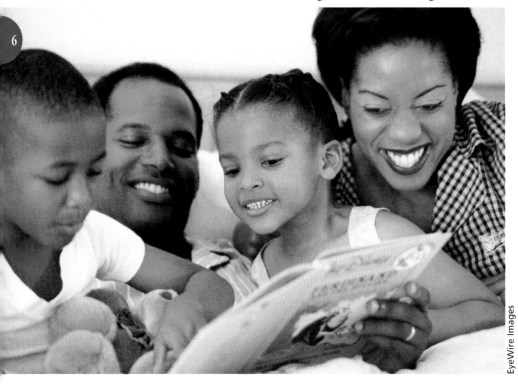

EyeWire Images

6

–isn't it about time we started looking for alternative solutions? Conventional medicine uses drugs as the answers to these disorders. However, the long list of side effects that accompany these solutions–ranging from dry mouth and nausea to seizures and changes to the reproductive system–are not acceptable to the informed parent.

Thankfully, there are other options–natural options–available to treat attention and learning disorders. Although solutions such as diet changes and nutritional supplements might not work as quickly as the drugs commonly prescribed for these problems, they do more than treat just the symptoms, like drugs do. There is hope for those who suffer from attention and learning disorders. There is hope for the families and teachers and communities who are affected by those who suffer. By eliminating toxins and changing the diet–and this includes the all-important essential fatty acids–you will not only treat the disorder causing the unpleasant symptoms, but you can work to prevent the disorders from manifesting themselves in the first place.

I receive lots of telephone calls, letters and emails from parents of children with learning disorders and from adults coping with their own learning difficulties. Their questions are always important to their personal concerns. But they all share a common interest. They are always eager to know more about why fatty acids are important for health in general and particularly for brain function. I always enjoy explaining the wonders of the human body to them!

One mother sent a thank you letter for the wonderful changes a fatty acid supplement had brought to her son and as a result her family. She said the changes in concentration and the ability to control his outbursts were just small examples of the delightful effects. He is now just a "normal" kid. She then asked if I could provide any information on fatty acids because she wanted to pass on all the benefits of her findings to other families "who also need HELP! Thank you! Thank you! Thank you!"

If you or your child suffer from an attention or learning disorder, you probably have tried a number of drug treatments already. It's time to try the permanent, healthful treatments described in this book. Not only will you experience relief from your disorder, but also from the side effects of drugs.

Natural solutions do more than just treat the symptoms, like drugs do.

If you are planning a family or have young children, give them the best chance for avoiding these disorders by taking the advice outlined here–your whole family will benefit!

What are Attention and Learning Disorders? . .

Attention-deficit disorder (ADD), attention-deficit hyperactivity disorder (ADHD), dyspraxia and dyslexia are closely linked attention and learning disorders. These four conditions are the main learning disabilities that handicap the progress of many children through school. For some, the condition tends to subside at puberty, but for most it continues throughout life.

Symptoms of Attention-Deficit Hyperactivity Disorder

Babies

- Extreme restlessness, crying, poor sleep patterns
- Difficult to feed
- Constantly thirsty
- Frequent tantrums, head banging or "rocking" the crib

Children

- Poor concentration and brief attention span
- Weak short-term memory
- Normal or high IQ but under-performs at school
- Physically active more often: always on the go or moving around
- Impulsive and fearless: doesn't stop to think before speaking or acting
- Poor coordination, for example, when tying shoelaces, using a pencil or playing ball games
- Inflexible personality: uncooperative, defiant and disobedient
- Lack of self-esteem: has problems making friends
- Sleep and appetite problems

Adults

- Most of the symptoms exhibited in childhood remain
- Employment might be difficult because of relationship problems and poor memory
- Antisocial behavior can become so extreme it can lead to trouble with the law or substance abuse

Children with ADHD are typically what most people call "hyperactive." They are excessively impulsive, destructive, distracted easily, restless and forgetful; can't sit still or listen, have difficulty organizing and completing tasks and have problems sleeping.

Nearly all children are overactive and inattentive at times, but the behavior of hyperactive children is extreme and completely disruptive to them and their families.

Children with ADD behave similarly to children with ADHD in that they have difficulty concentrating and focusing their attention, but the hyperactivity element is absent or minimal–they do not appear as restless as children with ADHD.

Dyslexic people have great difficulty reading and writing even though they have normal or above-average intelligence. They sometimes see and write words, letters or numbers in reverse and they have difficulty distinguishing similarities and differences among words.

Attention and learning disorders tend to run in families.

Dyspraxic people appear clumsy and uncoordinated. They have difficulty in planning and carrying out manual tasks requiring coordination, such as catching a ball.

People with these conditions might not have all the symptoms of the disorder and there are different degrees of severity for each symptom. Some individuals have more than one condition at the same time.

In addition, the conditions tend to run in families; a family could have one child with dyslexia, another with ADHD and another with dyspraxia.

Children often develop means of coping with their

EyeWire Images

9

symptoms and are able to lead productive lives with minimal difficulty. But sometimes, the disruptive nature of the conditions continues throughout life, making it more difficult for adults with these disorders to maintain successful careers, family life and community involvement. Statistics show, unfortunately, that higher rates of alcoholism, drug abuse and unlawful behavior exist in adults with ADHD. Considering the number of people afflicted with this or similar conditions, one can imagine the impact on families and on society in general. The consequences of going through life undiagnosed and without proper treatment can be devastating for people with these disorders and for those around them. That's why it's so important to recognize the problem early and start natural treatment right away.

Diagnosing the Disorders . . . .

Recent estimates indicate that 3 to 5 percent of school-aged children are suffering from attention-deficit hyperactivity disorder and surveys using broader definitions have increased that to 17 percent. Boys are more commonly affected than girls: in 1995, 18 to 20 percent of boys in grade five in two cities in the United States were reported to have ADHD and as a result were being treated with psychostimulant medications. The same year, a similar report said that 561,000 patients in Canada had been diagnosed with attention-deficit disorder. ADD support groups indicate that as many as 50 percent of children with ADD are never diagnosed, so the real numbers could be even higher.

Diagnosing ADD or ADHD is not an easy task and should be done in consultation with a qualified health-care professional. Diagnosis is based on the duration and degree of

Boys are more commonly affected by attention and learning disorders than girls are.

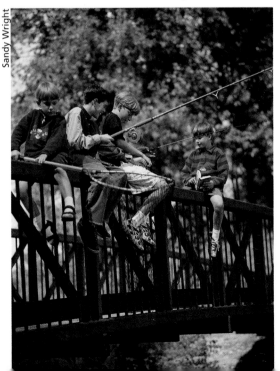

Sandy Wright

disruption that a child's condition causes to normal life–theirs and the lives of their parents, siblings, teachers and classmates. Symptoms must be present before age seven and must have persisted for at least six months to be considered attention-deficit disorder.

Most practitioners use one of two checklists of behavior to diagnose ADHD. One of these is found in the American Psychiatric Association's Diagnostic and Statistical Manual of Mental Disorders, fourth edition. The other is a tool called the Conners' Parent-Teacher Rating Scale, a questionnaire that lists a number of behaviors, including excitability/impulsivity, failure to finish tasks, worrying more than others, quarrelsomeness, and having frequent ailments such as headaches, etc. These are rated on a scale of 0 to 3 and a combined score of 15 or greater indicates that the child has ADHD.

Diagnosis usually includes a review of the child's personal and family history as well as physical and psychological assessments. However, your opinion as a parent is also extremely valuable. No one knows your child better than you do. If you feel uneasy with a particular diagnosis, then get a second opinion. Remember that you are your child's advocate and any diagnosis and subsequent treatment regimen can have future consequences.

Despite the use of these checklists, the condition is easy to misdiagnose. In fact, a survey of 800 school children in the US found that teachers were more likely to consider children who drink caffeine-containing beverages to be hyperactive than those who do not drink them. In addition, naturopathic doctor Eric Jones, author of the book *Alternative Medicine*, estimates that at least 50 percent of children labeled as having ADD have been misdiagnosed. Following the misdiagnosis is usually a prescription for drugs.

Learning and attention disorders are easy to misdiagnose.

11

A Word From the Publisher

Parents have two choices for treatment. Either they choose the "naturopathic" way, meaning nutrition-oriented natural medicine; or they choose the orthodox (allopathic) way, which involves pharmaceutical, chemical medicine. Most often the choice is influenced by the practitioner being consulted. Fortunately, parents do have a choice and it's the purpose of this book, as with all titles published in this series of Natural Health Guides, to provide education and information that will help in the decision-making process. As the proverb says: "Knowledge is Power."

–Siegfried Gursche

Standard Orthodox Treatments
for ADD and ADHD . . . .

The typical treatment for ADD and ADHD involves a combination of counseling and medication. Counseling may help sufferers learn how to control their tempers and improve their listening skills, problem-solving abilities and decision-making processes. Medications are also used to modify behavior. These include psychostimulants such as Ritalin® (methyl-phenidate) and Dexedrine® (dexamphetamine) to reduce impulsivity and improve concentration; antidepressants such as Prozac® (fluoxetine), Tofranil® (imipramine), Norpramin® (desipramine), Pamelor® (nortriptyline), Wellbutin® (bupropion) and Ludiomil® (maprotiline) to alleviate distractibility and relieve anxiety; and amphetamines such as Adderall®.

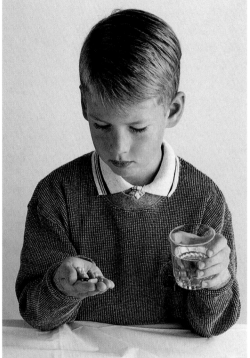

Typical treatment for ADD and ADHD involves drugs to modify behavior.

The use of methylphenidate has risen consistently since its introduction. The US Food and Drug Administration reports that sales of the product increased by nearly five times between 1990 and 1998 and roughly 90 percent of the drug produced globally is now consumed in the United States. Health Canada determined that the number of prescriptions written for methylphenidate in Canadian pharmacies rose from 138,000 in 1990 to 652,000 in 1997. Canada is the second-largest user of Ritalin. One study estimated that in 1995 nearly 1.5 million children between ages 5 and 18 were taking the drug. More recent reports show the sale of methylphenidate to be leveling off, but sales of amphetamines showed a three-fold increase between 1995 and 1997.

Drug treatments can be effective for relieving ADD/ADHD symptoms. In fact, experts report that psychostimulants can suppress symptoms in roughly 80 percent of people diagnosed with the conditions (meaning they don't work for 20 percent of patients). Unfortunately, this apparent success comes at a price, both financial and physical. Drugs are expensive; some of those mentioned can cost several dollars for a daily dose, amounting to hundreds of dollars per year. More importantly, these types of medications produce a number of unwanted–and unnecessary–side effects that are often as bad as the condition itself.

Drugs Cause Side Effects

The most common side effects of antidepressants include dizzy spells, dry mouth and urinary retention. Norpramin and many of the other antidepressants mentioned can cause more serious conditions such as tremors, seizures, skin rashes, nausea, vomiting, loss of appetite, altered liver function and changes to the reproductive system. Some people taking Norpramin have experienced serious irregular heartbeats and this has caused the sudden death of more than one child–it's certainly not worth the risk.

The list of common side effects of Ritalin includes nervousness, sleep disturbances, decreased appetite, dizziness, drowsiness and headache. Nausea, vomiting, abdominal pain, blood pressure changes, rapid heart rate, skin rashes and fever also can occur. In some cases, weight loss during prolonged therapy–to the point of causing stunted growth in some instances, muscle cramps, tics, and psychotic episodes (including hallucinations and depression) have been reported. Fortunately, there are gentler, more natural solutions.

Recently, many scientists have expressed concerns about the safety of using stimulant drugs since there is little information about their effects on the body after years of use. What long-term effects do they have on the nervous system, the reproductive system or the

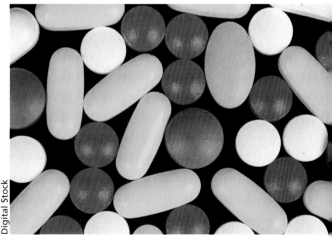

Digital Stock

The side effects of the drugs prescribed for attention and learning disorders are often as bad as the condition itself.

13

aging process, and do they cause cancer? Since most users of these drugs are children, and since they have to keep taking the drugs to keep symptoms at bay, these are important questions.

One study completed by the National Toxicology Program in the United States showed that doses equivalent to just two and a half times the maximum recommended dose of methylphenidate for humans did cause cancer in mice. The Food and Drug Administration agreed that the product might have the potential to cause cancer, although it pointed out that it does not cause cancer in rats and that mice might not be good predictors of cancer-causing abilities in humans. But is it worth the risk?

Why not consider the food your child is eating? Alternative treatment to the risks stated above are nutritional treatments. If it sounds simple, it's because it is simple. Diet can and will make a difference in your, or your child's, condition as can a whole range of non-drug treatments. It takes patience and dedication, however, the diet and lifestyle changes required to successfully treat an ADD sufferer will also benefit the entire family and in turn the society as a whole.

Diet Makes a Difference . . . .

A recent report by the Center for Science in the Public Interest reviewed the findings of twenty-three reliable studies to determine the impact of food dyes and/or ordinary foods on the behavior of children with ADHD and related problems. Some of these studies compared typical diets to ones that were specially designed to exclude various additives and other substances known to promote hyperactivity, such as caffeine. Others fed children diets devoid of potential irritants and then intentionally introduced things that typically caused reactions. (This is called a "challenge test.") These were blind studies, which means that the children, and everyone involved in evaluating the children's response, were unaware of what type of food was being eaten. This enabled the researchers to obtain unbiased results. Some of these studies clearly indicated that certain food substances can have an impact on a child's behavior.

Nine of the twenty-three studies included only children with ADHD. Eight of these nine studies reported that some of the

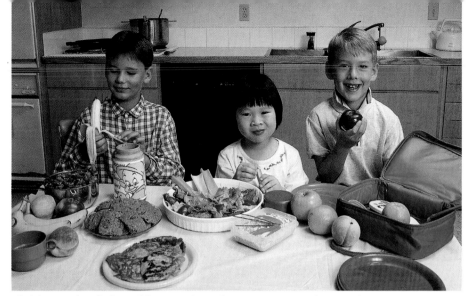

children either behaved better when they were eating diets without additives or got worse when they ate the irritating substances.

Diet *can* make a difference to people with ADD/ADHD, but anticipate subtle and possibly slow changes rather than dramatic and near immediate effects like those seen with drug treatments. Changes may be slower than with drugs; however, results are lasting and side effects non-existent.

The results of a healthful diet are effective and lasting.

What Causes ADD and ADHD? . . . .

There isn't one simple or obvious cause for either ADD or ADHD; however, since the most obvious place to look for alternative solutions for these problems is at potential causes, let's look into what factors contribute to ADD/ADHD.

Since learning disorders are particularly prevalent in Western society, it's only logical to look to our lifestyle for possible causes and triggers. Possible contributors are our dietary habits–eating processed, refined and preserved foods high in artificial additives, salt, sugar and artificially hardened fats (as found in margarine, shortening, hydrogenated oils, and in processed and junk foods) and low in nutrient content. Our daily living patterns, with less emphasis on traditional family structures and more energy given to hectic work schedules, giving us less time to spend with our loved ones, are also suspect. Others blame frequent use of television and video games that promote development of short and/or intermittent bursts of attention.

Scientists generally assume that the primary cause appears to be genetic (inherited). However, the possibility that these conditions are inherited does not mean you have no control over whether you or your child develop them. Other contributing factors, which could be considered triggers, include nutrition, food and environmental allergies, environmental contaminants, increased and repeated use of antibiotics and possibly physical problems such as spinal column misalignment.

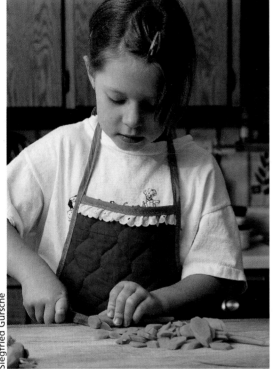

Siegfried Gursche

What we consume *can* have an impact on behavior.

Is Food to Blame?

We know that people who are prone to developing heart disease because of their genetic makeup can reduce their risk by changing their diet, reducing stress and exercising regularly. In the same way, someone genetically predisposed to ADD/ADHD may be able to alter the progression or manifestation of the condition by controlling environmental influences, such as diet.

It is completely reasonable to think that what we consume can have an impact on behavior. In fact, this has been proven time and time again and continues to be proven throughout daily modern living. A perfect example is alcohol. We all know that someone's behavior changes drastically after four or five drinks, and we know how good that first "kick" of caffeine feels in the morning, and how it can wake us up. So it is possible that certain components in food could be responsible for other behavioral changes.

Dr. Benjamin Feingold, an allergy specialist in San Francisco, made the first reports to this effect, in the mid-1970s. He found that 30 to 50 percent of hyperactive children improved when placed on a diet free of artificial colors and flavors, and substances called "salicylates," which occur naturally in many fruits. Twenty years of research investigating the impact of dietary components on behavior disorders followed.

What About the Environment?

Environmental contaminants are another possible source of difficulty for people with learning disorders. These contaminants include everything from chemical cleaners and building products that emit noxious substances into the air, to insecticides, pesticides and heavy metals that contaminate our air, food and water. They also can include mold spores that accumulate in poorly designed or older buildings. This particular problem is currently plaguing schools and other public buildings in many areas.

Studies have shown that children perform poorly on tests taken at school following application of floor cleaners and insecticides. Clearly, the easiest way to eliminate this problem is to avoid using these irritating substances. However, complete protection from exposure is practically impossible so certain safety measures should be considered. These include ensuring that ventilation ducts in

Exercising regularly and breathing fresh air contribute to a strong immune system, which adds protection from environmental influences.

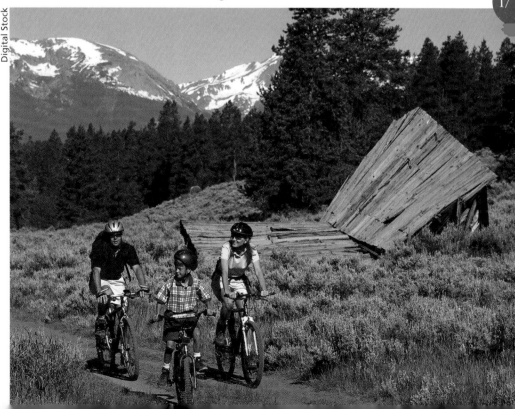

buildings are cleaned frequently, and the installation of air filtering or purifying systems. These steps could help remove unwanted materials from the air and ensure a healthier environment.

Ensuring that you or your child have a healthy immune system will also serve as protection from environmental influences. Eating a whole foods diet, getting a sufficient amount of sleep, exercising regularly and breathing fresh air all contribute to a strong immune system.

Antibiotics: Another Possible Culprit

Antibiotic use is another possible contributing factor in learning disorders. Repeated and prolonged use of antibiotics can kill the friendly bacteria that are supposed to live in our bodies. These micro-organisms are responsible for producing some of the nutrients we need, such as vitamin K, and for preventing other organisms from invading our bodies. Antibiotics kill these natural protectors. This can allow other harmful organisms (pathogens) to grow and flourish in our bodies once the antibiotic treatment is stopped (or even before). One of these pathogens is a yeast called *Candida albicans*. If it gets out of control, it can grow happily in our intestines, vagina and lungs and is normally controlled by our native bacteria. It can cause numerous symptoms, including anxiety, fatigue, irritability, headaches, hyperactivity, poor appetite and sleep disturbances.

Bacterial pathogens also can grow in the intestines and numerous different kinds have been found growing in the digestive tracts of children with ADD. Bad micro-organisms can contribute to a condition called "leaky gut." (Believe it or not, "gut" is the medical word used to describe the digestive tract.) That's when spaces develop between the cells that line the intestine, or the cells become less able to prevent the transfer of partially digested food from inside the gut to surrounding tissue. When partially digested food invades the system it can trigger an immune response because the body identifies the material as foreign and tries to destroy it. This situation can contribute to the development of allergies and can make you feel weak and ill.

One way of ensuring that yeast and bad bacteria do not invade our systems is to avoid antibiotic use so that our internal friendly bacteria colonies stay healthy. If you must use antibiotics, be sure to eat foods that contain friendly bacteria such as natural, live-culture yogurt, kefir, sauerkraut and miso. In addition, dietary supplements are available that contain these good bacteria, which include *Lactobacillus acidophilus* and *Bifidobacteria*. Treatment with these supplements should begin as soon as the antibiotic is completed.

Another way to ensure that *C. albicans* in particular cannot gain a foothold is to starve it. *C. albicans* feeds mostly on foods containing sugar, or that are converted to sugar in the body, such as candy, fruit and processed white flour. Eliminating these and other sources of sugar from the diet will prevent the yeast from growing and multiplying rapidly and will allow time for the friendly bacteria to become re-established. Infection with *C. albicans* and other micro-organisms can be diagnosed and treated successfully. Elimination of these pathogens should be one of the first priorities of someone with ADD or ADHD.

For more information on friendly intestinal bacteria, read *Friendly Bacteria* by Dalton Moore, *alive* Natural Health Guide #18, 2000).

Chiropractors report improvements in patients following treatment to realign the top of the vertebra in the neck.

Spinal Misalignment

Another, less talked about and perhaps less understood, factor contributing to learning disorders is spinal column misalignment. Some chiropractors have reported improvements in patients following treatment to realign the top vertebra in the neck. Misalignment of this bone places pressure on the brain stem and interferes with transmission of nerve impulses from the brain to the body and vice versa. This type of adjustment is called "atlas subluxation adjustment." Another type of adjustment, called "craniosacral therapy," adjusts the brain and the spinal cord. This reduces unwanted pressure that could be caused by incorrect positioning so that nerve impulses can travel more freely. Both of these therapies are drug-free and noninvasive.

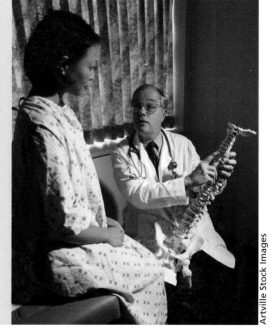

Artville Stock Images

Treatment and Prevention, Naturally . . . .

The options available for treating and preventing ADD and related conditions include a whole range of non-drug treatments. Selecting an appropriate treatment should be considered carefully. Working with a naturopath, or medical doctor who is supportive and knowledgeable about natural alternatives, can help. Many of these approaches are time consuming and can place great demands on parents and entire families to institute dietary and lifestyle changes. But most people find the rewards well worth the inconvenience. Besides, diet and lifestyle changes will benefit your whole family, not just the ADD sufferer.

The first move towards enhanced well being is eliminating possible aggravating factors, including allergenic foods, food additives, yeast infections and environmental contaminants.

An appropriate water filtration system will help remove wastes from the body.

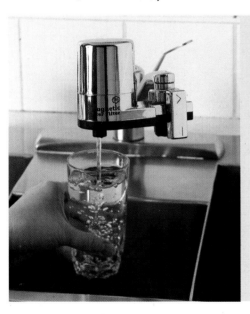

Detoxification

Detoxifying the body is one type of decontamination procedure that should be considered. This can be achieved using a number of herbal preparations and vegetable juices and by drinking lots of purified water.

Our drinking water can contain many harmful contaminants, including heavy metals such as lead; pesticides, herbicides and nitrates that have leeched from the soil; added ingredients such as fluoride compounds; and harmful bacteria or other pathogens. These substances should be removed from your water supply using an appropriate water filtration system. Drinking one to two liters of purified water every day will help remove wastes from your body and will replenish water losses.

You can make vegetable juices at home with a juicer starting with organically grown produce, including carrots, beets, celery, greens or any other desired ingredient. Alternatively, prepared vegetable juices are available at many health-food stores. These should be consumed in place of meals for three to four days to detoxify your system. Some practitioners recommend this procedure once a month to enhance the digestive system.

Dietary Management

Once aggravating infections and environmental and body contaminants have been eliminated, the next course of action should be to alter your child's diet. This can be one of the most challenging aspects of a natural approach to the treatment of attention and learning problems. You might have to change your entire family's diet to benefit one family member suffering from ADD or other behavioral or learning disturbances.

Avoid Additives

Start by eliminating food additives. Those identified as aggravating factors include artificial colors, flavors and preservatives. Many artificial food dyes are derived from coal tar—not something we should be eating! They reduce the ability of nerves and muscles to respond to signals from other nerves.

Avoid These Food Additives	
Substance	**Additional Information**
Flavors	
Monosodium glutamate (MSG), E621 Europe	Chinese food, flavor enhancers, canned soups, canned meat spreads, dry soup bases, prepared frozen foods, beef and chicken stock, packaged noodle and sauce mixes, vegetable juices
Preservatives	
Butylated hydroxy anisol (BHA), E320 Europe	Cookies, potato chips and other fatty snack foods, many highly processed bakery goods, refined (supermarket) oils
Butylated hydroxy toluene (BHT), E321 Europe	Cookies, potato chips and other fatty snack foods, many highly processed bakery goods, cereal packaging, refined (supermarket) oils

21

Potassium nitrate	Processed and packaged meats such as hot dogs and luncheon meats, smoked meats
Sodium benzoate, E211 Europe	Processed and packaged meats such as hot dogs and luncheon meats, smoked meats
Sodium nitrate, E251 Europe	Processed and packaged meats such as hot dogs and luncheon meats, smoked meats
Sodium nitrite, E250 Europe	Processed and packaged meats such as hot dogs and luncheon meats, smoked meats
Sulfur dioxide	

Salicylates and Phenolic Compounds

As I mentioned earlier, Dr. Feingold first identified salicylates as aggravating factors. Salicylates are the material from which Aspirin is made and are found in many foods, as listed below.

Avoid Foods Containing Salicylates	
Almonds	Nectarines
Apples	Oranges
Apricots	Peaches
Berries	Peppers (bell and chili)
Cherries	Plums
Cherry bark	Potatoes
Cloves	Prunes
Coffee	Raisins
Cucumbers and pickles	Tangerines
Currants	Tea
Eggplant	Tomatoes
Grapes	Willow bark
Mint and mint flavoring	Wintergreen and oil of wintergreen

Phenolic Compounds

Compounds made from salicylates, along with other similar materials produced naturally in the body, are called phenolic compounds. These substances appear in larger-than-normal amounts in the urine of people with autism–another learning/communication disorder–and to a lesser extent in the urine of people with attention and behavior problems. Phenolic compounds also can originate from incompletely digested proteins from milk and wheat, organic acids produced by "bad" micro-organisms growing in the intestine and other abnormal body processes.

Phenolic compounds are normally neutralized in the body by a particular enzyme. An enzyme is a protein molecule that is made in the body that acts like a catalyst (provided that you've got the right gene that codes for the protein). In other words, it helps to make a chemical reaction take place, for example, to change one thing to another, join things together or break things apart. In this case, it adds a sulfate group onto the phenolic compounds and enables them to be carried out of the body. Tests have shown that more than half of autistic children have either a deficiency in this enzyme or their enzyme is faulty, meaning that phenolic compounds build up in their systems. So it makes sense to avoid eating salicylates because they get made into phenolic compounds, resulting in even more of the harmful substances being present in the body.

The Feingold Diet

The Feingold diet recommends first eliminating from the diet all artificial colorings, flavorings, sweeteners (acesulfame-K, aspartame, saccharin, sucralose), some preservatives (BHA, BHT, TBHQ) and all foods containing salicylates. A complete list of ingredients to be avoided can be found on the Feingold website: www.feingold.org. Although there is not yet concrete scientific evidence confirming that flavorings, sweeteners or preservatives affect behavior and learning, many parents have found that eliminating these ingredients has helped their children. Salicylates and colorings, on the other hand, have been investigated and their effects reported in a number of studies.

If you do not see an improvement within two weeks of eliminating these substances, then there could be other chemicals or foods that are contributing to the problem. For example, allergies to certain foods can aggravate the condition. Remember that everyone is different, so some foods could cause difficulties for some people and have no effect on others. Foods that commonly cause allergic reactions include wheat, eggs, milk, chocolate, corn and soybeans. True food allergies can really only be identified

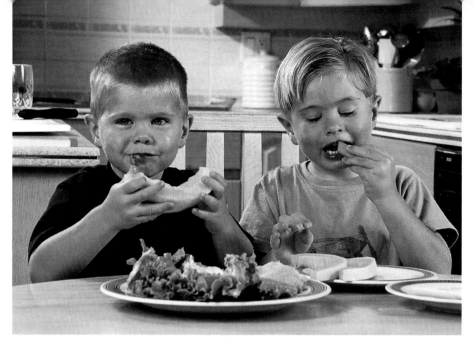

Eliminate all artificial colorings, flavorings, sweeteners and preservatives from the diet.

through diagnosis, which could include allergy testing and/or elimination diets.

Elimination diets involve restricting the suspected food from the diet and observing the child's behavior. These diets should be tried while also restricting additives and salicylates. After two weeks, the suspected food should be reintroduced to the diet (challenge test). If there is a drastic change in the child's behavior, then a food allergy or sensitivity is likely. The challenge test should not be attempted without the supervision of a qualified health-care provider. If an allergy is severe, the reaction could be life threatening.

Is it Really an Allergy?

It's important to know the difference between a food allergy and a sensitivity or intolerance to certain foods. A food allergy involves a rapid response by the immune system when the offending food is eaten. This can cause hives and swelling of tissue in the mouth and throat and can be so severe that the person goes into anaphylactic shock, which can lead to death if not treated immediately. A familiar example of this is the severe peanut allergy seen in some people.

Food sensitivities are more common than food allergies. They do not involve a drastic or immediate reaction by the body when the substance is eaten. They are not as dangerous, but even so they can be debilitating. Symptoms of food sensitivities include gas, bloating, heartburn, abdominal pain, diarrhea or constipation, nasal congestion, migraine headaches and leg pains.

If eliminating food additives, salicylates and food allergens and sensitivities doesn't work, the Feingold diet recommends restricting corn sugar (glucose and dextrose), corn syrup, monosodium glutamate (MSG), hydrolyzed vegetable protein and sodium nitrite (found in lunch meats and other processed meats). These recommendations are based on observations reported by parents.

Beyond these recommendations, a severely restricted diet–the "few-foods diet"–might improve behavior. This diet should be attempted for long periods and only in consultation with a qualified dietician to ensure that your child gets all the necessary nutrients. The few-foods diet excludes all the previously eliminated foods and substances, plus caffeine, chocolate, corn products, dairy foods, eggs, nuts, oranges and grapefruit, soybean products and wheat. This diet is so restrictive that it is actually easier to define what the child *can* eat: fresh meat and poultry, any vegetable except corn and soy foods, fruits and fruit juices (including pineapple and pear; excluding orange and grapefruit), rice and oats. If an improvement is noted after two weeks, then one eliminated food can be reintroduced at a time to determine which foods can be tolerated.

So Long, Sugar

Something else you should eliminate from your child's diet is sugar in all its many forms. This is because too much sugar can cause a variety of problems, many of them associated with hyperactivity and attention problems.

Sugar ...
- leads to malabsorption of protein and calcium and other minerals.
- slows growth of good intestinal flora and feeds yeast.
- causes the pancreas to work overtime to create more insulin.
- causes unstable blood sugar levels.
- decreases immune system function.

25

Sugar can cause a variety of problems associated with hyperactivity and attention disorders.

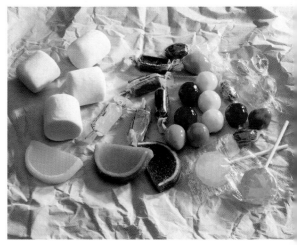

Sugar has been shown to decrease one's ability to concentrate, and destructive, aggressive and restless behavior increases with increased sugar consumption. Obviously, this will contribute to ADD symptoms.

One of the problems with sugar is that it causes unstable blood sugar levels, leading to hypoglycemia, which is another common trigger for ADD/ADHD. Low blood sugar levels cause the body to release adrenaline, which can cause hyperactivity and other ADHD symptoms. Other contributors to hypoglycemia are not eating often enough, skipping meals, not eating enough protein and complex carbohydrates and poor digestion.

For valuable information read *Health Hazards of White Sugar* by Lynne Melcombe (*alive* Natural Health Guides #22, 2000).

Correcting Nutritional Deficiencies

A number of researchers have identified nutritional deficiencies in children with ADD and learning disorders. Correcting these deficiencies sometimes can produce an almost immediate improvement in mental function in these individuals.

Some important minerals for people with ADD are iron, copper, calcium, magnesium and zinc. These last three are called the "sedative minerals." A high salt intake can reduce their levels in your body and can lead to hyperactive symptoms.

Correcting nutritional deficiencies can improve mental functioning.

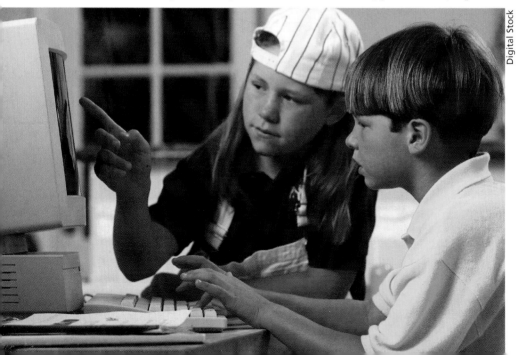

Digital Stock

Calcium and magnesium are also reduced by too much phosphorous, found in soda pop and red meat. Zinc prevents the nervous system from over-reacting to stress. Refined foods are low in zinc and stress depletes zinc stores, so zinc deficiency is common in the Western world.

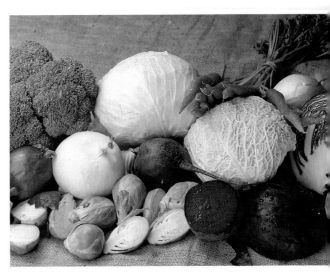

Iron deficiencies can cause a decreased attention span, decreased persistence and decreased voluntary activity. Iron supplementation increases the ability to concentrate, decreases fatigue and improves mood. Note that anemic people absorb lead more readily. Copper deficiency can develop after prolonged or recurring infections. The commonly used antibiotic penicillin also decreases copper stores.

Take advantage of the enzymes found naturally in raw foods.

Some nutritional deficiencies are due to an inability to properly digest food rather than a lack of certain nutrients in the diet. Therefore, even though you might be eating a nutritionally complete diet, you show signs of dietary deficiencies. You might experience other problems as well. For example, you could have symptoms associated with a leaky gut because the undigested food in your intestines helps feed unwanted pathogens that damage your intestinal lining.

Some experts recommend taking digestive enzymes to enhance the body's ability to absorb and use food properly. These enzymes are similar to those produced in our pancreas and other digestive organs and to the ones found in some raw foods. They include lipases, which split fat molecules; amylases, which digest starch; and proteases, which help break down proteins. If poor digestion is suspected, digestive enzymes might be recommended. Alternatively, it might be useful to take advantage of the enzymes found naturally in some foods. Raw foods are easier to digest because they can be partially digested by their own enzymes. Cooked foods, in contrast, do not contain any active enzymes because heat destroys them. Eat more raw food!

For more information read *Digestion: Your key to vibrant health* by Ken Babal (*alive* Natural Health Guides #25, 2000).

Herbal Treatments

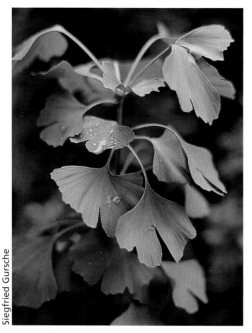

Siegfried Gursche

Ginkgo biloba can enhance memory function and increase ability to concentrate.

Ginkgo biloba is probably the herbal product recommended most frequently to enhance brain function. Its usefulness in relieving symptoms of aging, including memory loss, has been studied. It also has been reported to enhance memory function in youngsters and to increase their ability to concentrate and focus their attention, so it could help your ADD child.

Herbal remedies can be used to detoxify your system, enhance your immune system and improve circulation to your brain to ensure a good supply of nutrients and removal of toxic compounds. Many herbs are recommended in the scientific literature for these purposes.

Grape Seed and Pycnogenol

A product with action similar to Ginkgo biloba is grape seed, and a mixture of substances derived from it, as well as the bark of the French maritime pine called pycogenol. Its first recorded use in North America was by a group of French explorers trapped in the ice-filled Saint Lawrence River in 1534. When the sailors started to develop scurvy because of lack of vitamin C, the Native Americans recommended they drink a tea made from pine bark and leaves. That simple remedy saved the men from certain death. Four hundred years later a French scientist determined that the tea contained a powerful mixture of antioxidant substances that could provide protection to the body similar to vitamin C. Eventually, a better source of pycnogenol was discovered in grape seeds. Today, grape seed and pycnogenol are used for many conditions where improved circulation and antioxidant protection is required. This is particularly useful in ADD because it simultaneously helps nourish and protect the brain. In addition, pycnogenol has been shown in a six-week clinical study to improve vision, including vision in the dark and recovery from glare. The significance of this observation will become clear when I discuss polyunsaturated fatty acids in relation to learning disorders.

Detoxifying herbs include psyllium husk powder (which aids in elimination), garlic, milk thistle, parsley, red clover, stinging nettle, alfalfa, sage, dried hawthorn (fruit and flowers), burdock root, birch leaves, verbena and cat's claw tea. Cat's claw also enhances the immune system, helps reduce inflammation and regulates digestion so it is an effective means of combating problems associated with a "leaky gut."

Siberian ginseng is recommended as a tonic for children at doses of 100 to 200 milligrams of concentrated root extract per day. This herb also can be taken as a dry powder (1 to 1½ grams daily in two or three divided doses) or as an alcohol-based extract (4 to 5 milliliters in two divided doses). The product should be used for four to six weeks followed by two weeks without treatment before resuming the medication.

Other herbal products that have been studied for use in ADD/ADHD include catnip, thyme, chamomile, lemon balm, licorice root, hops, lobelia, passionflower, skullcap, rosemary, wood betony, mullein, St. John's wort, beet root, lemon grass, hibiscus and peppermint. Some of these have sedative qualities and are aimed at reducing the hyperactive components of ADHD.

You may want to talk to a herbalist or trained Natural Products Advisor in a health food store to get some suggestions for mixing up some herbs for a tasty herbal tea. Sweetened with honey, a tea, whether hot or cold, can be drunk several times a day, replacing cola drinks, which have a negative effect on those with ADD.

Dramatic results have been shown with valerian root extract. It calms the nerves with an action that is exactly the opposite of

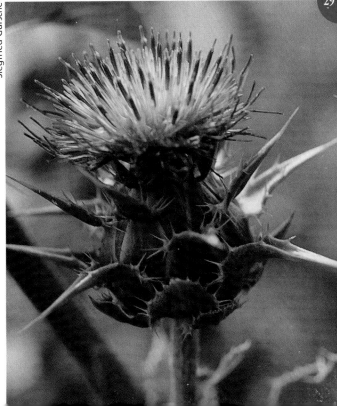

Siegfried Gursche

Detoxifying herbs, such as milk thistle, enhance the immune system, reduce inflammation and regulate digestion.

caffeine, which stimulates. Once valerian wears off it leaves no lasting effect. The extract should be mixed with juice as per the package directions and taken two to three times per day.

Supplements

The dosages recommended below are for adults. The recommended dose for teenagers between 12 and 17 years of age is three-quarters of the recommended amount. Children between six and twelve should use one half the dose and those under six, one quarter the adult dose.

Supplement	Suggested Dosage
Minerals	
Calcium	As directed on the label, at bedtime
Chromium	200 mcg daily
Copper	0.5-1 mg daily
Magnesium	As directed on the label, at bedtime
Zinc	5-10 mg daily
Vitamins	
Vitamin B complex	50 mg 3 times daily
Vitamin B$_3$ (niacin)	100 mg daily (do not exceed 300 mg daily from all sources)
Vitamin B$_5$ (pantothenic acid)	100 mg daily
Vitamin B$_6$ (pyridoxine)	50 mg daily
Vitamin C	1000 mg 3 times daily
Other Substances	
Brewers' yeast	Begin with ¼ tsp daily and increased to recommended label dose
Gamma-aminobutyric acid (GABA)	750 mg daily
L-cysteine	As directed on the label
Quercetin	As directed on the label

If a lack of certain nutrients in the diet is the probable cause of a deficiency, the problem can be corrected easily with dietary supplementation. In fact, providing vitamin and mineral supplements to children with ADD can enhance their performance even when there is no measurable deficiency, so this avenue is well worth investigating. Follow the advice of your health care provider concerning dosages and use with other medications and be sure to ask about any precautions that may be recommended specific to your needs.

In addition to the nutrients listed below, some specialists also recommend lecithin, proanthocyanidins, glutamine, bee pollen and specific fatty acids called long-chain polyunsaturated fatty acids, which are discussed in the next section.

Essential Fatty Acids

What follows in this section of the book is very important information. It may sound technical, but bear with me as I explain it in simple terms as well.

Long-chain polyunsaturated fatty acids (LC-PUFAs) are made from two special nutrients called essential fatty acids, which are found in the food we eat and are also natural components of our bodies. They are the building blocks for many of the fatty acids that make up the membranes in our cells.

Essential fatty acids are a crucial part of a healthful diet.

31

There are only two essential fatty acids (essential meaning we can't exist without eating them), but there are many fatty acids that can be made in the body starting with these parent fatty acids as building blocks. The two essential fatty acids are the omega-3 fatty acid (alpha-linolenic acid) and the omega-6 fatty acid (linoleic acid). We must eat these two fatty acids as part of a healthy diet because our bodies cannot make them. Alpha-linolenic acid is found in flax oil and, to a lesser extent, in dark-green leafy vegetables. Linoleic acid is found in great abundance in many seeds and nuts, and consequently in the oils processed from these. However, the processing method (known as refining) destroys the valuable

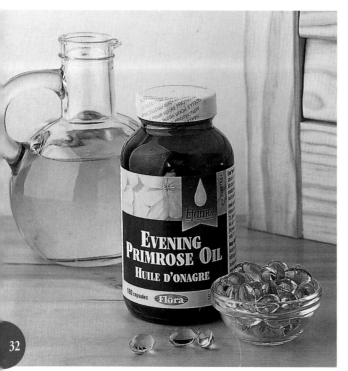

essential natural form. What results is an oil with harmful trans fatty acids. So, when I talk about vegetable oils containing essential fatty acids, I'm referring to the unrefined, cold-pressed oils usually found in health food stores only.

Once inside our bodies, linoleic acid is used to make other fatty acids including gamma-linolenic acid (GLA) and arachidonic acid. In the same way, alpha-linolenic acid is converted to fatty acids such as docosahexaenoic acid (DHA).

The process of converting one fatty acid to another is called metabolism; the

Efamol's evening primrose oil is one of the most popular sources for gamma-linolenic acid (GLA).

workers on this processing line are called enzymes. Some of the enzymes on this line don't always work the way they should. This interferes with the metabolism process and sometimes certain fatty acids are not produced as efficiently as they should be. Some of the fatty acids that might not be made include arachidonic acid and DHA. These fatty acids are the long chain polyunsaturated fatty acids (LC-PUFAs) mentioned earlier, and they make up a large part of the brain and eyes. In fact, the brain is about 60 percent fat and a high proportion of this fat is made with the fatty acids DHA and arachidonic acid. DHA is also extremely important for vision. If there are not enough of these fatty acids being made in the body, then the brain and eyes might not function properly.

Gamma-linolenic acid (GLA) is the first fatty acid that is made from linoleic acid on the processing line. Unfortunately, the enzyme that converts linoleic acid to GLA is usually the one that is not doing its job. That enzyme is delta-6-desaturase (D6D). So if GLA isn't produced, then neither is arachidonic acid. But if you eat GLA, then it is easier for your body to make arachidonic acid.

There are few nutritional sources of GLA, therefore it's best to take it as a supplement. Nowadays, one of the most popular sources for GLA is evening primrose oil. There are many brands, but almost all of the clinical trials to date have been conducted with the brand Efamol, which stands for "Essential Fatty Acids Molecules." For more information read *Evening Primrose Oil* (*alive* Natural Health Guide #6, 2000).

The mother of a child with ADD told me a very sad story about her dear son who was extremely hyper, very annoying, not doing well in school, not able to join any sports because he always had to win, was often angry and upset, was very difficult and was not much fun to be around. She also told me he was a very bright child, but no one including his own sister and brother wanted to play with him because if he didn't get what he wanted there

Supplementing the diet with a specific combination of essential fatty acids can have a dramatic effect.

would be a disaster. She then went on to tell me how supplementing his diet with GLA from evening primrose oil and DHA from fish oil changed his life and those around him.

He is now at the top of his class, in baseball and cubs, enjoys sharing, is very concerned about others, a real joy to spend time with, and the list goes on. She said he had only been taking a fatty acid supplement (Efalex) for two months, but they noticed a difference in two days. She said her family is totally happy with his change and no one is happier than he is. Her only concern was that she couldn't find a larger bottle of the product!

Fish Is Important

The enzyme that converts linoleic acid to GLA is the same one that converts alpha-linolenic acid to building blocks for DHA. So if alpha-linolenic acid isn't changed into these building blocks, then DHA isn't produced either. Fortunately, there are lots of good dietary sources of DHA. These include oily fish such as mackerel, salmon, tuna, herring and sardines. Unfortunately, many children don't like fish and even more concerning, more and more fish products are being identified as dietary sources of heavy metal contaminates such as lead and mercury. I personally question some of the testing that is done, however, it is worth trying to keep informed about.

Efamol, the company that manufactures evening primrose oil and other products containing fish oils that are used to treat ADD, tests every batch and the mercury content has never exceeded 0.01 mg per kg of oil (the lowest amount that can be detected by the analytical method). This means that if mercury were present at this detection limit then a daily dose would have less than 0.00004 mg. That's one million times less than the safe tolerance limit of 43 mg per day as set by World Health Organization themselves. As always, when purchasing any type of food or supplement, quality counts.

Oily fish, such as salmon, are good dietary sources of omega-3 fatty acid–docosahexaenic acid (DHA).

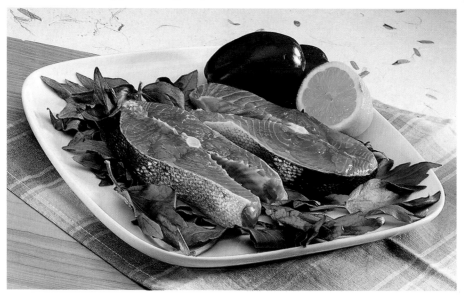

The Fatty Acid-ADD Connection

The idea that fatty acids could play a role in ADD and related conditions first came from observations reported by parents of children with ADHD. In 1981, Vicky Colquhoun and Sally Bunday, founders of the Hyperactive Children's Support Group in Britain, discovered this connection. As part of their early support activities, they completed a survey of a large population of hyperactive children, mostly boys, in West Essex, England, to determine what characteristics were common to hyperactive children. They found the following:

- Many hyperactive children had colic, eczema, asthma, allergies and repeated infections.
- Many of these children were zinc deficient.
- Most children complained of constant thirst.
- Certain food additives and salicylates could cause rapid behavioral deterioration.

These observations lead Colquhoun and Bunday to conclude that essential fatty acids were associated with the problem because of the following:

- The majority of children with ADHD are boys, and males need more essential fatty acids than do females, so a partial deficiency would be more apparent in boys.
- One of the first signs of essential fatty acid deficiency is thirst because lack of these oils in the skin allows water loss from the body through evaporation.
- Many children with eczema and allergies have problems metabolizing essential fatty acids.
- The enzyme delta-6-desaturate (D6D) requires zinc to work properly so zinc-deficient people cannot efficiently convert essential fatty acids to long chain polyunsaturated fatty acids (LC-PUFAs).
- Salicylates block the conversion of fatty acids to important regulatory substances called prostaglandins. LC-PUFAs and prostaglandins are important for brain function.

Colquhoun and Bunday concluded that hyperactivity might be due to a deficiency of essential fatty acids. However, they also recognized that the problem was unlikely to be caused by a dietary lack of these oils since often only one family member is affected even though the whole family eats the same foods. They speculated that the problem might be associated with a failure to convert dietary essential fatty acids (linoleic acid and alpha-linolenic acid) into LC-PUFAs (such as arachidonic acid and DHA). And since salicylates block the conversion of certain fatty acids to prostaglandins, this would help to explain the effects of salicylates as well.

Not Just Deficiency...Functionality

Controlled scientific studies have confirmed that it's not an essential fatty acid deficiency that is the problem; it is a functional essential fatty acid deficiency. That means that the body is not able to use the fatty acids that are supplied in the diet. So these children might be eating lots of linoleic acid and alpha-linolenic acid, but their bodies are not able to convert them to the long chain polyunsaturated fatty acids (LC-PUFAs) required for normal body function. So children with attention-deficit hyperactivity disorder (ADHD) have all the classic symptoms of essential fatty acid deficiency, even though they are eating enough of them.

The confirming study was done by Dr. Laura Stevens and Dr. John Burgess at Purdue University, Indiana. In their study, fatty acid levels were measured in children with ADHD (as determined using the Conners' Parent-Teacher Rating Scale). They also measured levels in children of similar ages who did not have ADHD (the control

Fatty acid functionality in the body is a factor in attention and learning disorders.

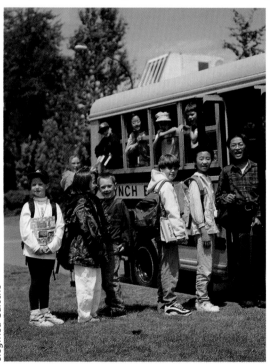

Siegfried Gursche

36

group). Parents evaluated signs of possible essential fatty acid deficiency, including extreme thirst, frequent urination, dry skin, dandruff and brittle nails. They also reported on headaches, stomach aches, diarrhea and constipation. A diet record was maintained for each subject to detect any differences in dietary intake between the control subjects and the children with ADHD that might account for differences in fatty acid levels.

> ### Unscientific Proof
> Sometimes just paying attention can mean the difference between successful treatment and years of struggle. Mothers of ADD children who start giving their kids specific fatty acids often write to me to say how much their childrens' teachers have noted changes in their children. One mom wrote about her son who was a high functioning autistic. She said his mood swings had decreased, he could sit for longer periods of time in school, he didn't get as frustrated anymore and he could concentrate better. She also said that his teacher was very impressed with the difference in him and that his recent report card was the best yet. She said she knew that fatty acid supplementation (GLA and DHA) made the difference because she ran out and he didn't take any for 8 days. On the third day he had to be removed from class because of his bad behavior. He became frustrated and generally miserable. When she realized what was missing, she quickly ran to the health food store and got some more. Within days, he was "back on track."

The researchers found that the ADHD children had lower-than-normal levels of DHA and arachidonic acid in their blood. There was no apparent difference between the diets of these children and the diets of the normal children. So it appears that either children with ADHD are not able to efficiently make fatty acids such as arachidonic acid and DHA from the essential fatty acids they eat or that they very quickly use what they do make. Either way, it leaves them without enough arachidonic acid and docosahexaenoic acid (DHA).

In a follow-up study, Drs. Stevens and Burgess found that children with higher amounts of omega-3 fatty acids such as DHA had better mathematics ability and overall academic ability. These same children were also less prone to behavior problems such as temper tantrums and to sleep problems. Those children with ADHD who had the lowest levels of DHA and arachidonic acid exhibited the most severe anxiety, impulsivity, hyperactivity and "conduct disorder." Children who had lower concentrations of the omega-6 fatty acids, such as arachidonic acid, seemed to have more colds and used more antibiotics. So it appears that the omega-6 fatty acids are important for the immune system as well as for brain function.

Breast Is Best

Research shows that children with ADHD were less likely to have been breastfed and if they were breastfed, it was for a shorter period than were children in the control group. A similar observation was noted in dyslexics by another researcher in the UK and so the biological link between these learning disorders was first proposed. That proposal was made by Dr. Jacqueline Stordy, who researched the role of nutrition in dyslexia; in 1995 she discovered that DHA could be important.

Dr. Stordy first noticed that in families with more than one person with dyslexia, those who had been breastfed the longest were the least affected by their dyslexia and in general their problems had become apparent later in childhood. As it turns out, breast milk is an excellent source of DHA, arachidonic acid and GLA. Therefore these fatty acids could provide a protective effect for children who have inherited the likelihood of developing the condition.

Children with attention-deficit disorder were less likely to have been breast fed.

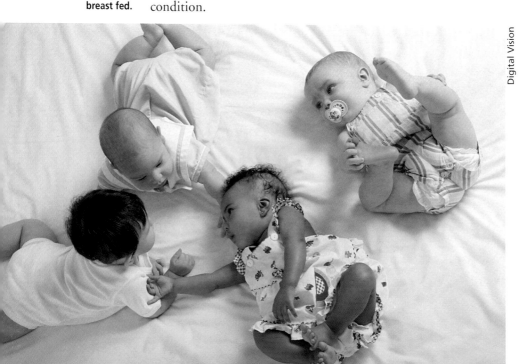

Digital Vision

Mothers need to eat more omega-3 fatty acid foods, such as salmon, mackerel, herring, sardines and flax seed oil. Add flax seed oil or freshly ground flax seeds to salad dressings, dips, soups, yogurt and quark, and vegetable juices.

Prevention Starts Before Birth

The cause of impaired fatty acid metabolism in children with ADHD and related conditions is still being investigated, but research indicates that modern lifestyles could be a factor, including the typical Western diet–high in saturated and processed fats, cholesterol and excessive alcohol, as well as stress and frequent viral infections. All these have been shown to slow or partially block the conversion of essential fatty acids to GLA, arachidonic acid and DHA. These effects can have an impact on a person's brain not only during childhood, but even before birth. Studies completed at the Institute of Brain Chemistry in England have shown that much of the selective

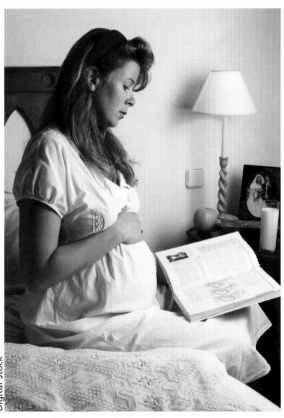

uptake of fatty acids by the brain takes place through the placenta during gestation and via breast milk in the first six months to one year of life.

Essential fatty acids are an important part of both the prenatal and postnatal diet of mothers.

In the early stages of pregnancy, fatty acids are needed for growth of the placenta. As the pregnancy progresses, further demands are made on the mother's fatty acid supply as the placenta and fetus grow. During the last three months of pregnancy, there is a rapid accumulation of DHA and arachidonic acid in the eyes and brain cells of the fetus. In fact, at this stage, the baby's brain increases four to five times in weight. So it is crucial that the mother has a supply of DHA and arachidonic acid sufficient to meet the needs of the fetus at this critical time of development.

It is also important to have a sufficient fatty acid supply during breastfeeding. During the first few months of life, the baby's nervous system continues to grow very rapidly and DHA and arachidonic acid play a very important role in this development. Breast milk provides the DHA and arachidonic acid the baby needs. However, there have been some studies showing that the LC-PUFA content of breast milk can vary widely from mother to mother. This is because it depends on her diet *and* on her ability to convert the essential fatty acids from her diet into LC-PUFAs. So it is important that the mother ensures an adequate intake of fatty acids, such as Efamol's clinically proven evening primrose oil.

All pregnant women should consume 1.5 percent of their dietary energy as essential fatty acids and LC-PUFAs. That equals about 3.6 grams per day for an average pregnant woman. Lactating mothers should eat 11 grams per day of essential fatty acids and LC-PUFAs since these vital nutrients are passed on to the baby through breast milk. If one was taking all of this as a dietary supplement, that would be about nine to ten 500 mg capsules of a highly polyunsaturated fatty acid like evening primrose oil and/or fish oil per day for a pregnant woman or 28 to 30 capsules per day for lactating mothers. Of course, you wouldn't want to take that much as a nutritional supplement because your daily food intake should provide you with some as well. These quantities of capsules have merely been provided to give you a practical idea of how much oil that would be.

A lot of research in recent years supports the need to supply adequate amounts of LC-PUFAs to the fetus and to infants to enable good visual and intellectual development. In 1998, two reports from the University of Dundee in Scotland showed that problem-solving ability in infancy could be enhanced by LC-PUFA supplementation. The researchers concluded that "since higher problem-solving scores in infancy are related to higher childhood IQ scores, supplementation with LC-PUFAs may be important for the development of childhood intelligence."

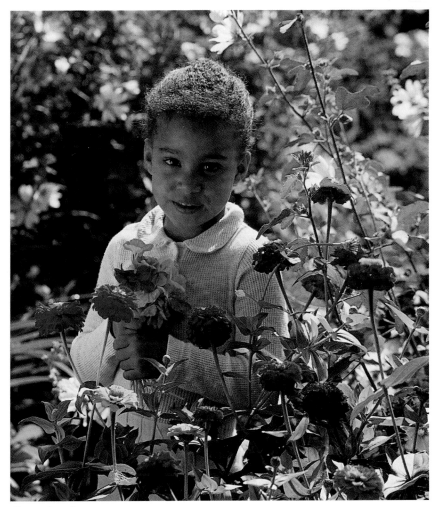

Conclusion . . . .

Research holds much promise for those afflicted with learning
disorders. Investigations in this area are ongoing and with the
future will come more solutions and methods of prevention. It is
already apparent that current natural approaches can be useful for
adults and children with an inherited tendency towards ADHD,
ADD, dyslexia and dyspraxia. In addition, much evidence suggests
that preventive measures can reduce these debilitating conditions
in our population. We can all help by putting our knowledge to
good use.

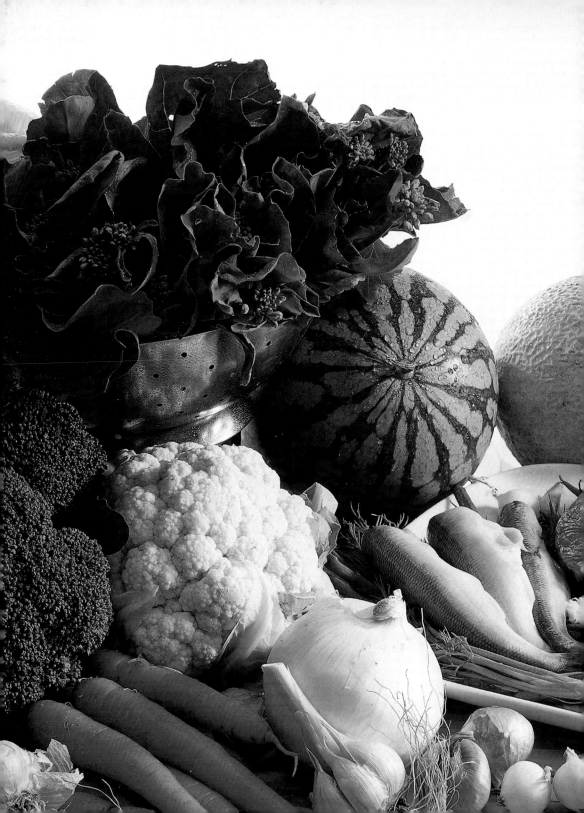

Revolutionary Health Books
alive **Natural Health Guides**

Each 64-page book focuses on a single subject, is written in easy-to-understand language and is lavishly illustrated with full color photographs.

New titles will be published every month.

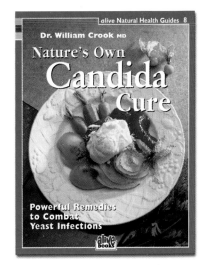

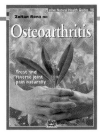
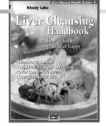

Series 1

Self Help Information

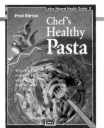
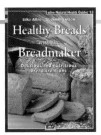

Series 2

Healthy Recipes

Great gifts at an amazingly affordable price
Cdn $9.95
US $8.95

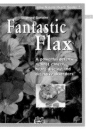
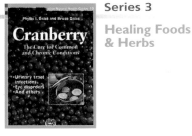

Series 3

Healing Foods & Herbs

alive **Natural Health Guides**
are available
in health food stores,
nutrition centers and
bookstores. For information
or to place orders please dial
1-800-663-6513

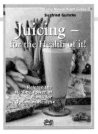
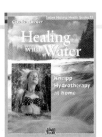

Series 4

Lifestyles & Alternative Treatments

alive books
Vancouver
Canada

references

Stordy, B. J. "Feeding the Brain...From Conception to Maturity."
ADD News. Vol. 2, no. 2 (1999): 14, 23.

Stordy, B. J. "Feeding the Brain...From Conception to Maturity."
Kentville, NS: Efamol Canada, 1999, audiotape.

Weintraub, Skye. *Natural Treatments for ADD and Hyperactivity.*
Pleasant Grove, UT: Woodland Publishing, 1997.

Willatts, P. et al. "Effect of Long Chain Polyunsaturated Fatty Acids
in Infant Formula on Problem Solving at 10 Months of Age." *The
Lancet.* Vol. 352, no. 9129 (1998): 688-91.

— et al. "Influence of Long Chain Polyunsaturated Fatty Acids on
Infant Cognitive Function." *Lipids.* Vol. 33, no. 10 (1998): 973-80.

www.addofoundation.org/info.htm
www.butterflymail.com
www.cspinet.org
www.feingold.org
www.maff.gov.uk/food/infsheet/1998/No156/156diet.htm
www.tnp.com

sources

for evening primrose oil and Efalex:
Efamol Canada Ltd.
35 Webster St., suite 103
Kentville, NS B4N1H4
(902) 678-2727

Efamol
Newmarket Ave., White Horse Business Park
Trowbridge, Wiltshire BA14OXQ
0 870 6060 128

for grape seed extract, ginkgo and pycnogenol:
Natural Factors Nutritional Products Ltd.
3655 Bonneville Place, Burnaby, BC
V3N 4S9
Phone: 1-800-663-8900
Fax: 1-800-663-2115

for water filter:
Teldon of Canada Ltd.
7432 Fraser Park Drive
Burnaby, BC V5J 5B9
Phone: (604) 436-0545
Orders: 1-800-663-2212
Fax: (604) 435-4862
E-mail: teldon@ultranet.ca

Remedies and supplements mentioned in this
book are available at quality health food stores
and nutrition centers.

First published in 2000 by
alive **books**
7436 Fraser Park Drive
Burnaby BC V5J 5B9
(604) 435–1919
1-800–661–0303

© 2000 by *alive* books

Book Design:
 Liza Novecoski
Artwork:
 Terence Yeung
 Raymond Cheung
Food Styling/Recipe Development:
 Fred Edrissi
Photography:
 Edmond Fong
 (except when credited otherwise)
Photo Editing:
 Sabine Edrissi-Bredenbrock
Editing:
 Sandra Tonn
 Donna Dawson

Canadian Cataloguing in
Publication Data

Nancy L. Morse, CNPA
 Attention-Deficit Disorder

(*alive* Natural Health Guides, 29
ISSN 1490-6503)
ISBN 1-55312-032-9

Printed in Canada

references

Al, M.D.M. et al. "Maternal Essential Fatty Acid Patterns During Normal Pregnancy and Their Relationship to the Neonatal Essential Fatty Acid Status." *British Journal of Nutrition.* 74 (1995): 55-68.

Alder, E.M. and J.L. Cox. "Breast Feeding and Post-natal Depression." *Journal of Psychosomatic Research.* Vol. 27, no. 2 (1983): 139-44.

Anderson, N. and H. Peiper. "ADD: The Natural Approach." Safe Goods. (1997). This is a book. It is published by a company called Safe Goods, East Canaan, CT, USA

Bell, R. and H. Peiper. "The ADD and ADHD Diet." *Safe Goods.* 1997.

Block, Mary Ann. "ADHD: A Demand for a Healthy Diet?" *Delicious! Your Guide to Natural Living.*

Brenner, RR. "Nutritional and Hormonal Factors Influencing Desaturation." *Progress in Lipid Research.* 20 (1981): 41-47.

Brown, D.J. *Herbal Prescription for Better Health.* Rocklin, CA: Prima Publishing, 1995.

Brush, M.G. et al. "Abnormal Essential Fatty Acid Levels in Plasma of Women With Premenstrual Syndrome." *American Journal of Obstetrics and Gynecology.* 10 (1984): 363-66.

Burgess, J.R. et al. "Long-chain Polyunsaturated Fatty Acids in Children With Attention-deficit Hyperactivity Disorder." *American Journal of Clinical Nutrition.* 71 (2000): 327-30.

Carter, J.P. "Gamma-linolenic Acid As a Nutrient." *Food Technology.* (June 1988): 72-82.

Chevallier, A. *The Encyclopedia of Medicinal Plants.* Montreal, QC: Reader's Digest Assoc., 1996.

Clandinin, M.T. et al. "Assessment of the Efficacious Dose of Arachidonic and Docosahexaenoic Acid in Preterm Infant Formulas: Fatty Acid Composition of Erythrocyte Membrane Lipids." *Pediatric Research.* Vol. 42, no. 6 (1997): 819-25.

Colquhoun, I. and S. Bunday. "A Lack of Essential Fatty Acids As a Possible Cause of Hyperactivity in Children." *Medical Hypotheses.* 7 (1981): 673-79.

Crawford, M. "The Role of Essential Fatty Acids in Neural Development: Implications for Perinatal Nutrition." *American Journal of Nutrition.* 57 (1993): 703S-10S.

Gazella, K.A. "Essential Fatty Acids and Learning Disorders." *International Journal of Integrative Medicine.* Vol. 1, no. 4 (1999): 27-33.

Gillis, M. Claire et al, eds. *Compendium of Pharmaceuticals and Specialties,* 33rd ed. Ottawa: Canadian Pharmacists Assoc., 1998.

Holdcroft, A. et al. "Changes in Brain Size in Normal Pregnancy." *Journal of Physiology.* 498 (1997): 54.1

Holman, R.T. et al. "Deficiency of Essential Fatty Acids and Membrane Fluidity During Pregnancy and Lactation." *Proceedings of the National Academy of Science.* 88 (1991): 4835-39.

Horrobin, D.F. "Essential Fatty Acids, Psychiatric Disorders and Neuropathies." In *Omega 6 Essential Fatty Acids: Pathophysiology and Roles in Clinical Medicine,* ed. D.F. Horrobin. New York: Wiley-Liss, 1990, pp. 303-19.

— and M.S. Manku. "Premenstrual Syndrome and Premenstrual Breast Pain (Cyclical Mastalgia): Disorders of Essential Fatty Acids (EFA) Metabolism." *Prostaglandins, Leukotrienes, and Essential Fatty Acids Reviews.* 37 (1989): 255-61.

Jacobson, M.F. and M.S. Schardt. *Diet, ADHD & Behavior: A Quarter Century Review.* Center for Science in the Public Interest, Washington, D.C.,1999.

Lutz, M. "Diet As a Determinant of Central Nervous System Development: Role of Essential Fatty Acids." *Archives of Latinoam Nutrition.* Vol. 48, no. 1 (1998): 29-34.

Lyon, M.R. "Healing the Hyperactive Brain." CHFA Expo West, 2000. Audiotape 000330-330.

Makrides, M. et al. "Are Long-chain Polyunsaturated Fatty Acids Essential Nutrients in Infancy?" *The Lancet.* 345 (1995): 1463-68.

— "Effect of Maternal Docosahexaenoic Acid Supplementation on Breast Milk Composition." *European Journal of Clinical Nutrition.* 50 (1996): 352-57.

— "Erythrocyte Docosahexaenoic Acid Correlates With the Visual Response of Healthy, Term Infants." *Pediatric Research.* Vol. 33, no. 4 (1993): 425-27.

Richardson, A. et al. "Abnormal Cerebral Phospholipid Metabolism in Dyslexia Indicated by Phosphorus-31 Magnetic Resonance Spectroscopy." *NMR in Biomedicine.* 10 (1997): 309-14.

Taylor KE and Richardson AJ. Visual function, fatty acids and dyslexia. Prostaglandins Leukotrienes and Essential Fatty Acids 2000 Jul:63 (½):89-93.

Richardson AJ and Ross MA. Fatty acid metabolism in neurodevelopment disorders: a new perspective on associations between attention-deficit/hyperactivity disorder, dyslexia, dyspraxia and the autistic spectrum. . Prostaglandins Leukotrienes and Essential Fatty Acids 2000 Jul:63 (½):1-9.]

Schardt, D. "Diet and Behavior in Children." *Nutrition Action Healthletter.* Vol. 27, no. 2 (2000): 10-11.

Stevens, L. et al. "Essential Fatty Acid Metabolism in Boys With Attention-Deficit Hyperactivity Disorder." *American Journal of Clinical Nutrition.* Vol. 62, no. 4 (1995): 761-68.

— "Omega-3 Fatty Acids in Boys With Behavior, Learning and Health Problems." *Physiology and Behavior.* Vol. 59, no. 4-5 (1996): 915-20.

Stordy, B.J. "Benefit of Docosahexaenoic Acid Supplements to Dark Adaptation in Dyslexics." *The Lancet.* Vol. 346, no. 8971 (1995): 385.

— "Dyslexia, Attention Deficit Hyperactivity Disorder, Dyspraxia-Do Fatty Acids Help?" *Dyslexia Review.* Vol. 19, no. 2 (1997).

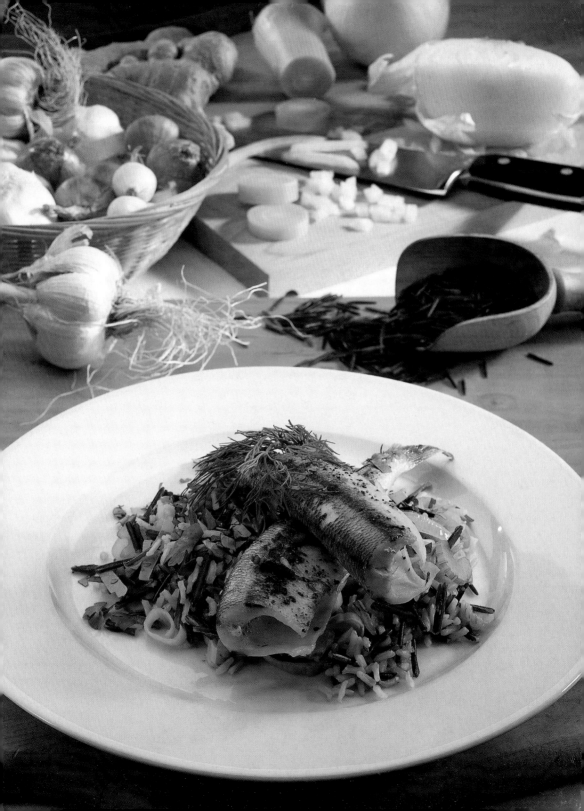

Red Snapper Wrapped in Rice Paper

Getting enough essential fatty acids in the diet is an important part of human nutrition. Fish is a good source of dietary DHA, the fat that is important for proper brain and eye function, particularly in growing children. Any kind of fatty fish is good prepared this way.

1 red snapper filet, ¼ lb (125 g), **cut in strips**

1 cup (250 ml) **carrots, julienned**

1 cup (250 ml) **snow peas, julienned**

1 cup (250 ml) **leek, julienned**

1 cup (250 ml) **celery, julienned**

1 cup (250 ml) **bok choy, chopped**

1 cup (250 ml) **Chinese cabbage, julienned**

2 tsp garlic, minced

1 tsp fresh ginger, minced

Pinch wasabi (optional)

1 tbsp toasted sesame seed oil

1 tsp sesame seeds

12 pieces rice paper, 8" rounds

2 tbsp extra-virgin olive oil

Reserve a bit of the carrots, snow peas and Chinese cabbage for garnish. Sauté fish, vegetables, garlic, ginger and wasabi in sesame seed oil for 5 to 7 minutes or until tender. Remove from heat, stir in sesame seeds and let cool.

Soak rice paper in warm water for 10 seconds. Place 2 pieces of rice paper directly on top of each other on a clean flat surface. Fill with 2 ½ tablespoons of the fish-vegetable mixture. Roll one end of the rice paper over the filling, tuck in the sides, and complete rolling. Sauté rolls in olive oil until golden brown on all sides. Serve garnished with julienned carrot, snow peas and Chinese cabbage.

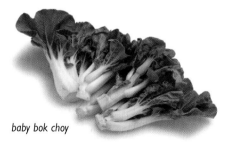

baby bok choy

> **Wrapping Tip**
> Use the double wrap to give more body and prevent the rice paper from breaking apart.

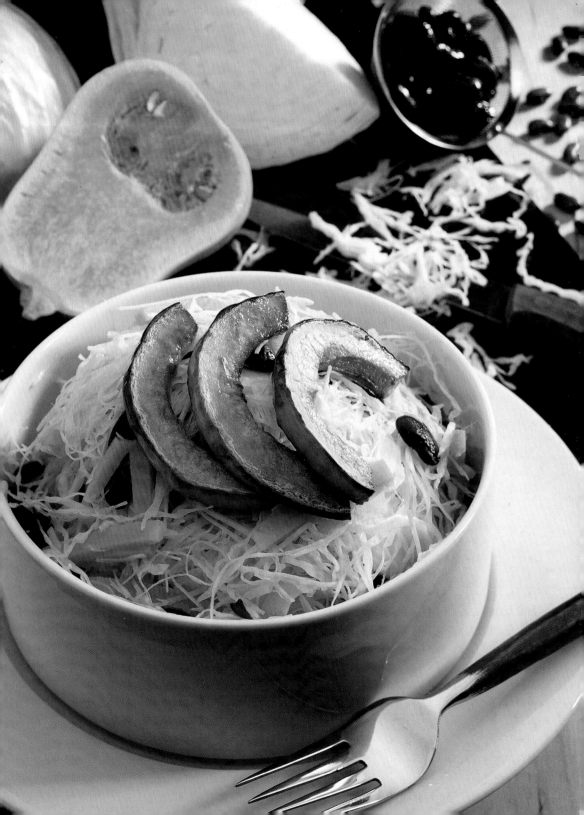

Cabbage-Bean Salad
with Roasted Squash

Correcting nutritional deficiencies in ADD sufferers can produce an almost immediate improvement in mental function. Cabbage supplies vitamins C, E, folic acid and other B vitamins, fiber and potassium. Squash is an excellent source of carotenoids, potassium, calcium and magnesium.

6 large wedges squash, skin on, cut ¼" (5 mm) **thick**

1 cup (250 ml) **squash, skin removed, cut in 3"** (8 cm) **strips**

2 cups (500 ml) **white cabbage, shredded**

1 cup (250 ml) **kidney beans, cooked**

1 tbsp extra-virgin olive oil

Herbamare, to taste

Dressing:

⅓ cup (80 ml) **pineapple juice**

3 tbsp walnut oil

1 tbsp green onion, chopped

Herbamare, to taste

Preheat oven to 375°F (190°C).

Brush squash wedges with olive oil, season with salt and pepper then roast in oven for 7 to 10 minutes until slightly golden brown.

Blanch squash strips for 3 to 4 minutes in a pot of boiling salted water. Drain and rinse with cold water.

In a bowl, whisk together all dressing ingredients then add the cabbage, beans and blanched squash; toss well.

Place salad onto plates, arrange roasted squash over top and serve.

Serves 2

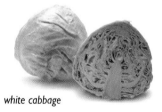

white cabbage

> ### Cooked Kidney Beans
> To cook kidney beans, first cover dried beans with water and soak overnight or at least 8 hours. Drain and cook in fresh water for 45 to 50 minutes or until soft.

> ### Vitamin B Boost
> You can also stir nutritional yeast into the dressing to supply B vitamins needed to support and strengthen the nerves.

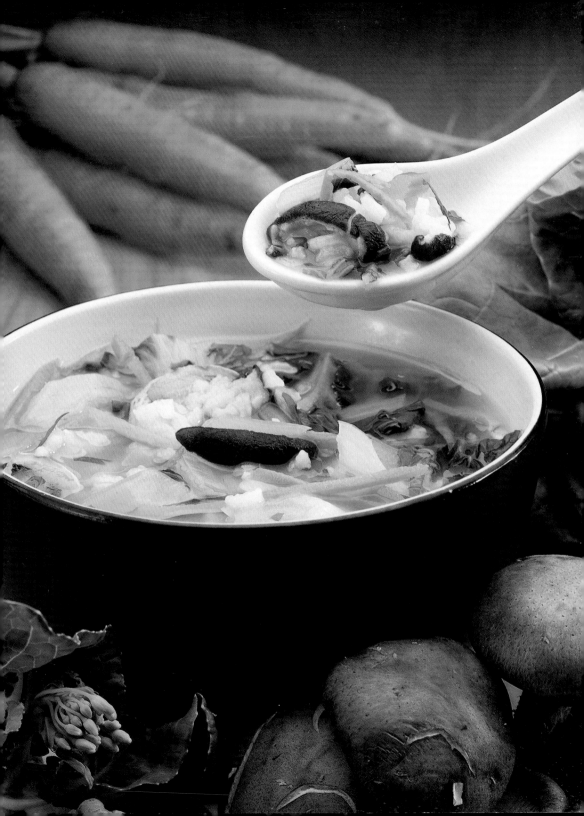

Rice Soup with Chinese Broccoli

Rice calms the nervous system and promotes mental health, supplying vitamins B and E, iron, amino acids and linoleic acid. Always choose nutrient-rich brown rice over white or parboiled varieties.

2 tbsp green onion, chopped

2 cloves garlic, minced

1 tsp fresh ginger, minced

1 cup (250 g) **Chinese broccoli** (gai lan)**, cut in 3"** (8 cm) **strips**

1 cup (250 ml) **leeks, chopped**

1 cup (250 ml) **shiitake mushroom, sliced**

1 cup (250 ml) **carrots, julienned**

1 cup (250 ml) **celery, julienned**

1 cup (250 ml) **siu choy, julienned**

2 tbsp extra-virgin olive oil

4 cups (1 l) **vegetable stock**

1 cup (250 ml) **brown rice, cooked**

1 tsp fresh cilantro, chopped

Herbamare, to taste

In a large pot, heat oil over medium heat and briefly sauté onion, garlic, ginger and all vegetables (except cilantro). Add vegetable stock and cook for 3 minutes or until vegetables are tender. Stir in rice, cook for 3 to 4 minutes longer then add cilantro. Remove from heat; let sit for 2 minutes. Season with Herbamare and serve.

Serves 2

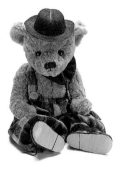

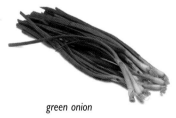

green onion

If your child prefers noodles to rice, substitute the brown rice for rice noodles.

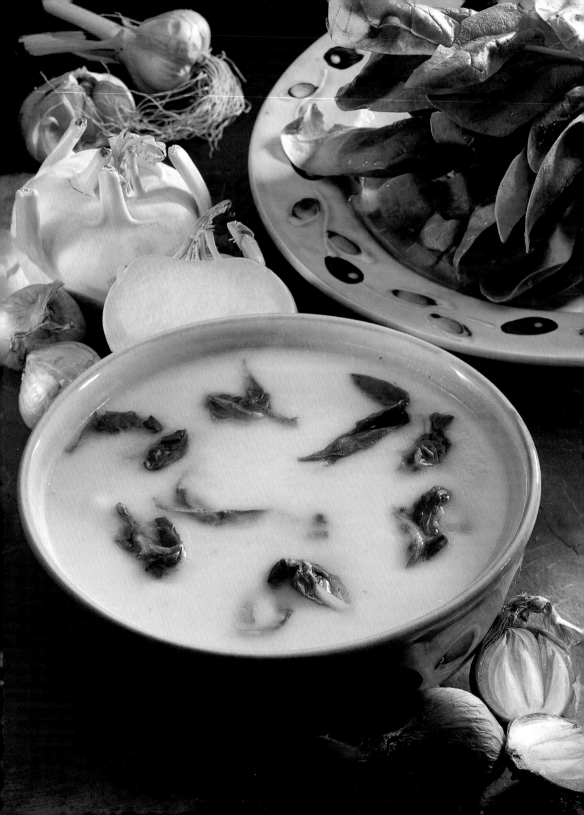

Spinach-Kohlrabi Soup

The combination of spinach and kohlrabi makes for a superior source of vitamin A, iron and calcium–all important nutrients for people with ADD.

1 lb (500 g) **baby spinach leaves**

2 cups (500 ml) **kohlrabi, peeled and cubed**

2 cloves garlic, minced

1 cup (250 ml) **white onion, minced**

¼ cup (60 ml) **celery, diced** (or celery root)

2 tbsp extra-virgin olive oil

2 cups (500 ml) **vegetable stock**

1 bay leaf

1 cup (125 ml) **rice milk**

Pinch vegetable salt

Bring 2 quarts (2 l) of salted water to a boil and blanch baby spinach for 15 to 20 seconds. Drain and rinse with cold water in order to stop the cooking and maintain the spinach's bright green color. Drain well and set aside.

In a large pot, heat oil over medium heat and sauté kohlrabi, garlic, onion and celery for 3 to 5 minutes. Add vegetable stock and bay leaf; cook for 10 minutes then stir in rice milk and simmer for 5 minutes longer. Remove from heat, pour into blender and blend until smooth. To make the soup velvety, strain it through a fine sieve. Transfer back to the pot, stir in blanched spinach and serve.

Serves 2

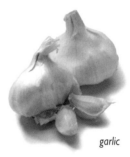

garlic

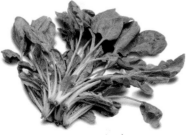

spinach

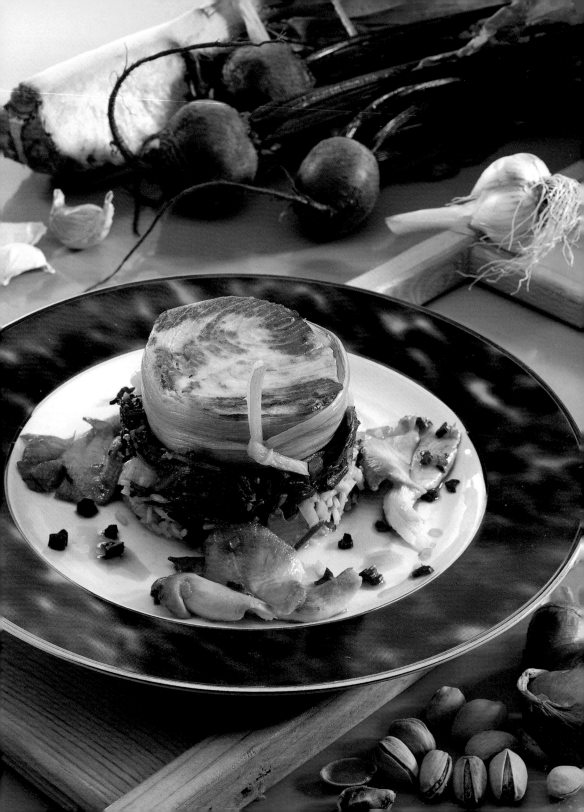

Tuna Sandwich with Bean Salad

Include fish in your family's diet as a source of the essential fatty acids important for brain function. The B vitamins found in nutritional yeast and green leafy vegetables support and strengthen the nerves.

Sandwich:

1 can white tuna in water

½ cup (125 ml) **onion, finely diced**

½ cup (125 ml) **celery, finely diced**

2 tbsp extra-virgin olive oil

4 leaves red leaf lettuce

1 ripe avocado

2 tbsp kefir

4 slices rye bread, toasted

Pinch Herbamare

To make the sandwich, rinse the tuna in the can several times with cold water, draining well. Place tuna in a bowl and break it into small pieces using a fork. Add onion, celery and oil; mix well. Spread toasted bread with kefir then assemble the sandwich, layering lettuce, avocado slices and tuna mixture.

To prepare the salad, blanch wax beans in salted boiling water for 5 minutes–no longer. Drain and rinse in cold water; drain well then cut the beans in half. Toss all salad ingredients together in a bowl and serve with the tuna sandwich.

Serves 2

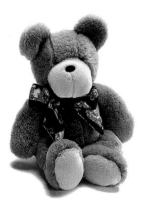

Salad:

1 cup (250 ml) **yellow wax beans**

1 cup (250 ml) **green wax beans**

1 tbsp fresh pineapple juice

2 tbsp extra-virgin olive oil

½ tsp nutritional yeast

1 tsp chives, chopped

1 cup (250 ml) **radicchio, julienned**

2 tbsp green onion, chopped

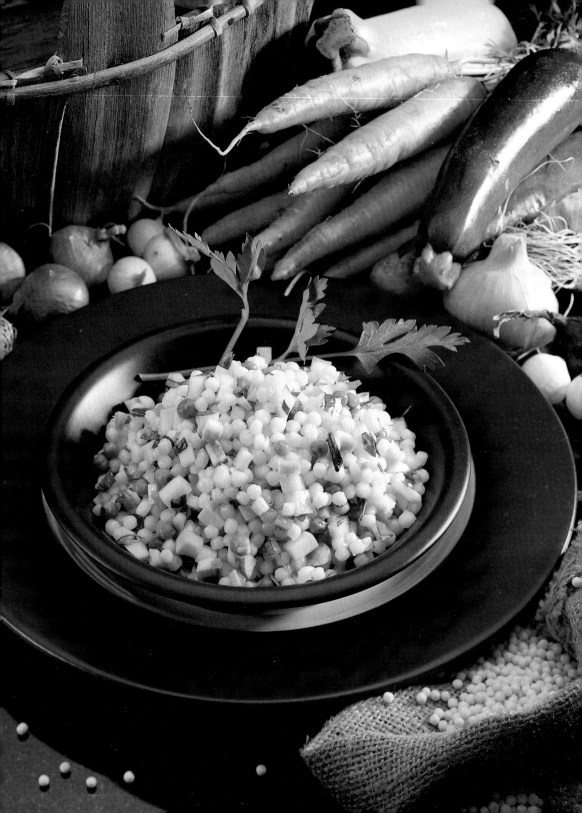

Israeli Barley Salad

Cultivated as far back as 9,000 years ago, barley has been traditionally eaten to increase mental alertness and physical strength. Hull-less barley is significantly more nutritious than pearl barley.

1 cup (250 ml) **barley**

1 cup (250 ml) **fresh green peas**

1 cup (250 ml) **carrot, finely diced**

1 cup (250 ml) **zucchini, finely diced**

1 cup (250 ml) **celery, finely diced**

1 cup (250 ml) **red onion, finely diced**

1 tbsp fresh parsley, chopped

2 cloves garlic, minced

1 tsp nutritional yeast

¼ cup (60 ml) **extra-virgin olive oil**

3 tbsp mango juice

Herbamare, to taste

Cook barley in salted water for 15 to 20 minutes. Drain and rinse in cold water. Drain well.

Blanch peas in salted boiling water for 2 minutes–no longer. Drain and rinse in cold water. Drain well.

Combine all ingredients in a large bowl. Cover and leave at room temperature for at least 2 hours before serving, in order for the flavors to incorporate.

Serves 2

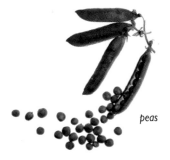

peas

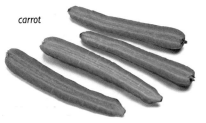

carrot

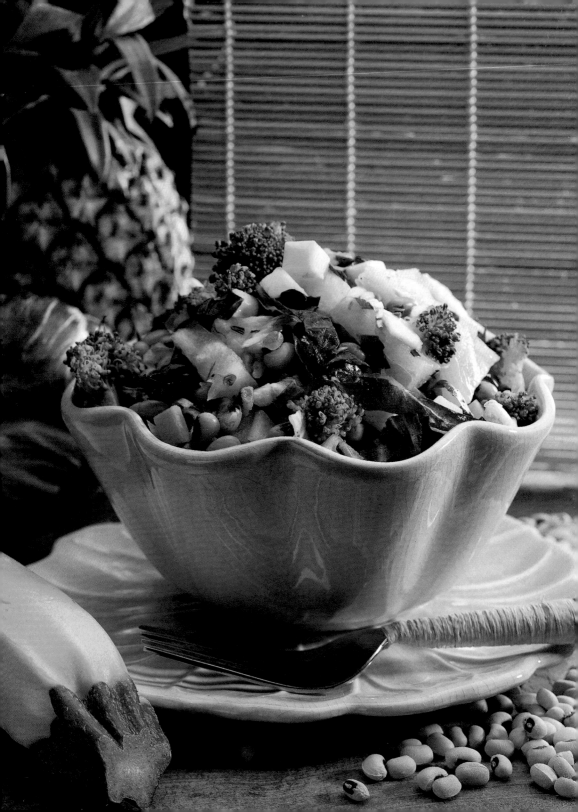

Pineapple-Broccoli Salad

Vitamin C from fresh raw vegetables aids the body in removing heavy metals. Nutritional yeast provides B vitamins, and adds a nice tangy flavor as well.

1 cup (250 ml) **fresh pineapple, diced**

1 cup (250 ml) **broccoli florets**

1 cup (250 ml) **black-eyed peas, cooked**

1 cup (250 ml) **zucchini, diced**

1 cup (250 ml) **radicchio, julienned**

¼ cup (60 ml) **white onion, julienned**

Dressing:

¼ cup (60 ml) **cold-presssed pumpkin seed, pistachio, extra-virgin olive or flax seed oil**

3 tbsp pineapple juice

2 tsp fresh Italian parsley, chopped

1 tsp nutritional yeast

Just rinse black-eyed peas, you don't need to presoak! Cook black-eyed peas in salted boiling water for 30 to 35 minutes or until soft.

In a large bowl, whisk together all dressing ingredients, add vegetables and black-eyed peas and toss well.

Serves 2

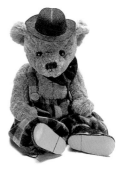

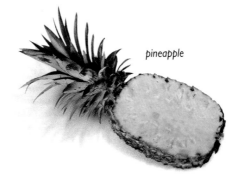

pineapple

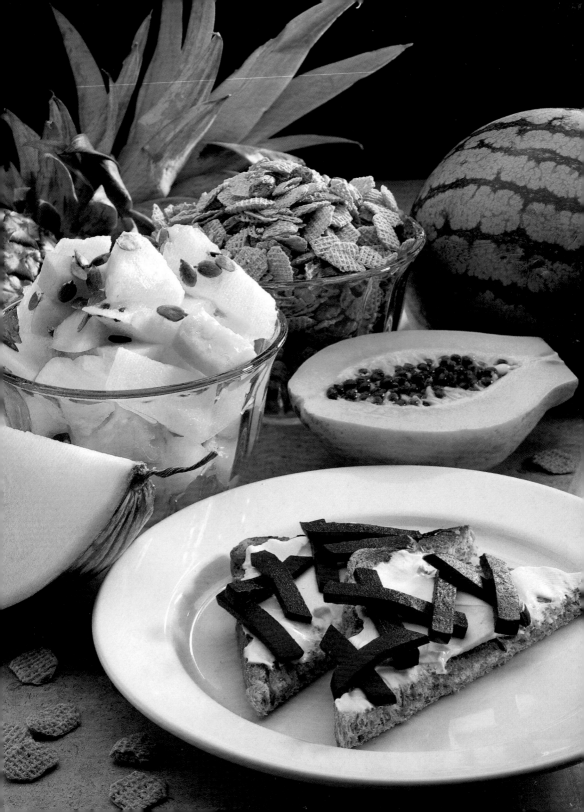

Red Beet-Kefir Breakfast

Breakfast is the most important meal for all of us, especially children, who require up to one-third of their daily nutritional needs to prevent a sudden drop in attention span around midmorning. For some reason, children love to eat beets, perhaps because it's fun to eat something that spreads such a bright color all over their hands and face. Beets contain significant amounts of calcium, iron and magnesium, and pumpkin seeds supply lots of zinc–important minerals for their calming effect on people with ADD.

½ **cup** (125 ml) **kefir**

2 **tbsp flax seed, pumpkin seed or walnut oil**

4 **slices rye bread, toasted**

½ **cup** (125 ml) **red beets, cooked** (recipe below) **and cut in strips**

2 **cups** (500 ml) **fresh fruit such as papaya, pineapple or watermelon**

2 **tbsp raw pumpkin seeds**

In a small bowl, combine kefir and oil. Spread toast with the kefir-oil mixture and place beet over top. Serve with fresh fruit sprinkled with pumpkin seeds.

Serves 2

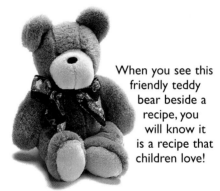

When you see this friendly teddy bear beside a recipe, you will know it is a recipe that children love!

Cooked Beets
In a large pot, combine 4 quarts (4 l) water and a small cinnamon stick; bring to a boil. Add 4 medium beets, sliced in ¼" (5 mm) rounds and simmer for 25 minutes or until tender. Drain and let cool. You can cook the beets a day ahead if you wish.

Treat ADD without the high cost of dangerous side effects. Choose natural foods.